THE
GOOD
ENERGY

COOKBOOK

365 DAYS OF WHOLESOME RECIPES TO HEAL YOUR METABOLISM, LOSE WEIGHT AND LIVE LONGER INSPIRED BY DR. CASEY MEANS' STUDIES

JADE BECKETT

THE
GOOD
ENERGY
COOKBOOK

365 DAYS OF WHOLESOME RECIPES
TO HEAL YOUR METABOLISM, LOSE
WEIGHT AND LIVE LONG! INSPIRED
BY DR CASEY MEANS' STUDIES

JADE BECKETT

TABLE OF CONTENTS

INTRODUCTION   7
Author's Philosophy   10

BREAKFAST
Sunrise Scramble   12
Omega Morning Muffins   13
Zesty Lemon Chia Pudding   14
Protein Power Pancakes   15
Avocado Toast Deluxe   16
Berry Bliss Smoothie Bowl   17
Sunrise Smoothie   18
Nutty Quinoa Porridge   19
Toasted Coconut Yogurt Parfait   20
Green Detox Twist   21
Golden Turmeric Oat Bowl   22
Cinnamon Apple Protein Waffles   23
Savory Spinach and Feta Muffins   24
Silky Matcha Yogurt Bowl   25
Sunrise Citrus Salad   26
Spicy Tomato Avocado Toast   27
Keto Blueberry Lemon Muffins   28
Smoked Salmon and Avocado Bowl   29
Pumpkin Spice Protein Oatmeal   30
Mediterranean Egg White Skillet   31

MAIN DISHES
Seared Tuna Pepper Steak   32
Lemon Herb Roasted Chicken   33
Spicy Shrimp Zoodle Bowl   34
Vegan Cauliflower Tacos   35
Thai Basil Beef Stir Fry   36
Grilled Portobello Mushroom Steaks   37
Mediterranean Chickpea Salad Bowl   38
Lemon Garlic Salmon Skewers   39
Butternut Squash and Black Bean Chili   40
Grilled Peach and Chicken Salad   41
Caribbean Jerk Turkey Bowl   42
Sesame Ginger Tofu Stir-Fry   43
Zesty Lime Fish Tacos   44
Herb Crusted Pork Tenderloin   45
Stuffed Bell Peppers   46
Pesto Zucchini Noodles   47
Garlic Lemon Scallops   48
Moroccan Spiced Vegetable Tagine   49
Thai Coconut Curry Shrimp   50
Rosemary Balsamic Beef Skewers   51
Savory Mushroom Risotto   52
Citrus Herb Grilled Salmon   53
Asian-Inspired Chicken Lettuce Wraps   54
Spiced Lamb Kebabs   55
Beef and Broccoli Stir-Fry   56

Quinoa Stuffed Tomatoes 57
Pan-Seared Cod with Citrus Salsa 58
Ratatouille with Baked Eggs 59
Spinach and Artichoke Chicken 60
Vegan Mushroom Stroganoff 61

SNACKS

Crunchy Chickpea Poppers 62
Zesty Lime Kale Chips 63
Sweet Potato Toasts 64
Nutty Fruit Energy Balls 65
Spiced Nut Mix 66
Greek Yogurt and Berry Parfaits 67
Cucumber Hummus Bites 68
Avocado Deviled Eggs 69
Tomato Bruschetta 70
Baked Apple Chips 71
Veggie Spring Rolls 72
Peanut Butter Banana Bites 73
Stuffed Dates 74
Cheesy Garlic Breadsticks 75
Roasted Garlic Edamame 76
Caprese Salad Skewers 77
Carrot Cake Energy Bites 78
Savory Olive Tapenade 79
Smoked Salmon Cucumber Rolls 80
Mini Bell Pepper Nachos 81

DESSERTS

Chia Lemon Raspberry Parfait 82
Coconut Mango Ice Cream 83
Dark Chocolate Avocado Mousse 84
Baked Cinnamon Apple Chips 85
Matcha Green Tea Panna Cotta 86
Walnut-Stuffed Baked Pears 87
Berry Yogurt Bark 88
Spiced Carrot Cake Squares 89
No-Bake Peanut Butter Bars 90
Zucchini Chocolate Chip Cookies 91

60-DAY MEAL PLAN

Tips for Success 93
Adjusting the Plan 94
Your Plan 95

INTRODUCTION

Welcome to The Good Energy Cookbook: 365 Days of Wholesome Recipes to Heal Your Metabolism, Lose Weight and Live Longer, a culinary journey designed to transform your health and revitalize your life. As a best-selling author and recognized expert in nutrition and weight loss, I've spent years exploring the powerful connection between what we eat and how we feel. Inspired by the pioneering research of Dr. Casey Means, this cookbook is more than just a collection of recipes—it's a blueprint for a vibrant, healthier future.

Each recipe in this book is crafted with one goal in mind: to harness the intrinsic power of food to optimize your metabolism, shed unwanted pounds, and extend your lifespan. The connection between diet and health is undeniable, and through Dr. Means' studies, we've gained invaluable insights into how certain foods can act as medicine, altering body chemistry in ways that promote healing and vitality.

In these pages, you'll find recipes that are not only delicious but are also tailored to boost your energy and metabolic health. From invigorating breakfasts to nourish your morning to nutrient-packed dinners that repair and rejuvenate your body overnight, each dish is designed to be as enjoyable as it is effective.

Whether you're a seasoned chef or a novice in the kitchen, these recipes will fit seamlessly into your daily life, guiding you towards better health with every bite.

This cookbook is also a testament to the power of personal responsibility. In today's fast-paced world, taking charge of your health is more crucial than ever. With every recipe, you're not just feeding yourself; you're consciously deciding to live better, longer, and with more vitality. It's about making informed choices, understanding the science of nutrition, and applying it in the most delicious way possible.

As we embark on this year-long journey together, remember that each recipe is a step toward a more energetic and fulfilling life. I invite you to cook your way through this book, embrace the science behind each meal, and feel the transformation within yourself. Let's reclaim our health, one delicious dish at a time.

Author's Philosophy

Hello, I'm Jade Beckett, and I welcome you to a chapter very close to my heart in this culinary journey we're undertaking together. My philosophy on food and health has been deeply inspired by the groundbreaking insights of Dr. Casey Means. In her compelling vision, she illustrates that the essence of our wellbeing hinges on our metabolic health—how effectively our cells generate and utilize energy. This revelation has not only influenced my culinary choices but also reinforced my commitment to the Mediterranean diet, a passion I'm eager to share with you.

Imagine a lifestyle where every meal you consume could potentially transform your health, reversing and preventing ailments ranging from the mildest discomforts like insomnia to severe conditions such as heart disease and diabetes. Dr. Means proposes that the "good energy" our cells generate is the cornerstone of such vitality. It's a concept that resonates deeply with me, as it aligns with the core principles of the Mediterranean diet—eating not just for survival, but for a vibrant, nourishing life.

Why the Mediterranean diet, you might ask? This diet, rich in fruits, vegetables, whole grains, and healthy fats, primarily olive oil, is celebrated not just for its deliciousness but also for its scientific backing in promoting longevity and reducing disease risk. Each meal under this diet is an opportunity to fuel your body with what I like to call 'premium energy sources.' These foods are minimally processed, close to nature, and deeply satiating—not just to your palate but to your cells.

The synergy between Dr. Means' insights and the Mediterranean diet is clear: both advocate for a return to whole, unrefined foods that our bodies are inherently designed to process. Foods rich in omega-3 fatty acids, such as fish and olive oil, nuts packed with antioxidants, and an abundance of fresh produce, provide our cells with the necessary tools to thrive and generate abundant good energy.

In this book, we explore not just recipes but a lifestyle that encourages a vibrant metabolism. Each recipe is crafted with ingredients that are proven to enhance metabolic health—foods that are as delightful as they are nourishing. My aim is to demystify the art of healthy eating, making it accessible, enjoyable, and fundamentally transformative.

Dr. Means also emphasizes the importance of understanding our unique biological makeup through modern tools and technologies. Just as she suggests, I encourage you to explore these options, to better understand your body's needs and how it reacts to different foods. This understanding has empowered me to select ingredients and recipes that best support my metabolic health, and I hope to pass on this knowledge to you.

Moreover, integrating simple movement into our daily routines, respecting our circadian rhythms, and occasionally challenging our bodies with natural elements like cold and heat can dramatically boost our metabolic efficiency. These practices are not just supplementary—they are foundational to building a lifestyle that embraces good energy.

As we navigate through each recipe and tip in this book, remember that we are not just feeding our stomachs but fueling our cells. We are stepping away from processed, energy-draining substances and embracing natural, energy-enhancing foods that Dr. Means champions and the Mediterranean lifestyle exemplifies.

Together, let's cook, eat, and live in a way that brings us closer to the vibrant health and good energy we all deserve.

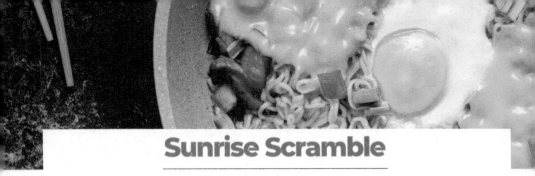

Sunrise Scramble

INGREDIENTS

- 4 large eggs
- 1/2 cup chopped bell peppers
- 1/4 cup chopped onions
- 1/4 cup spinach
- 2 tbsp milk
- Salt and pepper
- 1 tbsp olive oil

PREP. TIME: 10   SERVINGS: 2

DESCRIPTION

A vibrant, energizing egg scramble with fresh vegetables and herbs. Low in carbs and fats, perfect for a light start.

DIRECTIONS

1. Whisk the eggs with milk, salt, and pepper until well blended.
2. Heat olive oil in a non-stick skillet over medium heat.
3. Sauté onions and bell peppers until they are soft, about 3-5 minutes.
4. Add the spinach and cook until wilted, approximately 1-2 minutes.
5. Pour the egg mixture over the vegetables, stirring gently to combine. Cook until the eggs are set but still soft, about 3-4 minutes. Serve warm.

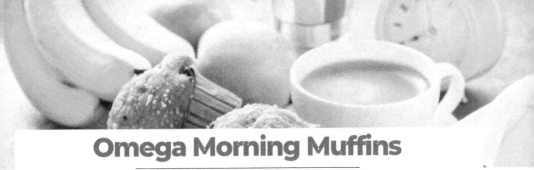

Omega Morning Muffins

INGREDIENTS

- 1 cup almond flour
- 1/2 cup ground flaxseed
- 1/4 cup walnuts, chopped
- 2 large eggs
- 1/4 cup honey
- 1 tsp baking powder
- 1 tsp vanilla extract
- 1/2 tsp cinnamon

PREP. TIME: 15

SERVINGS: 6

DESCRIPTION

Heart-healthy muffins packed with omega-3s from flaxseeds and walnuts. Low in carbs, high in protein and fiber.

DIRECTIONS

1. Preheat your oven to 350°F (175°C) and line a muffin tin with paper liners.
2. In a bowl, mix almond flour, flaxseed, baking powder, and cinnamon.
3. In another bowl, whisk eggs, honey, and vanilla extract until smooth.
4. Combine wet and dry ingredients and stir until just mixed. Fold in chopped walnuts.
5. Distribute the batter evenly among the muffin cups.
6. Bake for 20 minutes or until a toothpick inserted into the center comes out clean. Allow to cool before serving.

Zesty Lemon Chia Pudding

INGREDIENTS

- 1/3 cup chia seeds
- 1 1/2 cups almond milk
- 2 tbsp lemon juice
- Zest of one lemon
- 1 tbsp honey
- Fresh berries (for topping)

PREP. TIME:
15

SERVINGS:
2

DESCRIPTION

A refreshing and zesty pudding rich in fiber and protein, with a tang of lemon. Great for digestion and boosting energy.

DIRECTIONS

1. In a mixing bowl, combine chia seeds, almond milk, lemon juice, lemon zest, and honey.
2. Whisk thoroughly to prevent clumping.
3. Cover the bowl and refrigerate for at least 4 hours, preferably overnight, until the pudding has thickened.
4. Stir the pudding once more before serving. Adjust sweetness if needed.
5. Serve in bowls, topped with fresh berries for added vitamins and color.

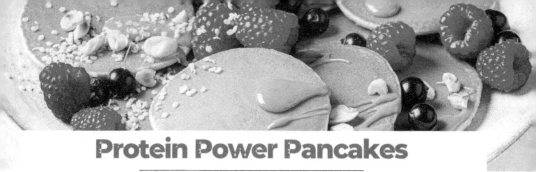

Protein Power Pancakes

INGREDIENTS

- 1/2 cup rolled oats
- 1/2 cup cottage cheese
- 4 egg whites
- 1 banana, mashed
- 1 tsp baking powder
- 1/2 tsp vanilla extract

PREP. TIME: SERVINGS:
10   4

DESCRIPTION

Protein-packed pancakes using cottage cheese and oats, keeping you full longer and aiding in muscle recovery.

DIRECTIONS

1. Blend the oats in a blender until they reach a flour-like consistency.
2. Add cottage cheese, egg whites, mashed banana, baking powder, and vanilla extract to the blender. Blend until smooth.
3. Heat a non-stick skillet over medium heat and lightly grease with cooking spray.
4. Pour 1/4 cup of batter for each pancake onto the skillet. Cook until bubbles form on the surface, then flip and cook the other side until golden, about 2 minutes per side.
5. Serve warm with a dollop of Greek yogurt or fresh fruit.

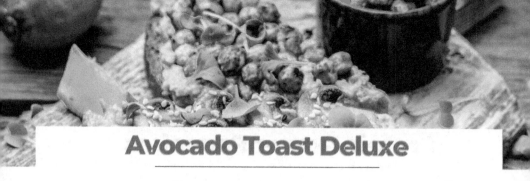

Avocado Toast Deluxe

INGREDIENTS

- 2 slices of low-carb bread
- 1 ripe avocado
- 4 radishes, thinly sliced
- 1/2 cup microgreens
- 1 tbsp lemon juice
- Salt and pepper

PREP. TIME: SERVINGS:
5   2

DESCRIPTION

A gourmet version of the classic avocado toast, topped with radishes and microgreens. Low-carb and rich in healthy fats.

DIRECTIONS

1. Toast the bread slices to your preferred doneness.
2. In a bowl, mash the avocado with lemon juice, salt, and pepper.
3. Spread the mashed avocado evenly on each slice of toast.
4. Top with sliced radishes and a generous handful of microgreens.
5. Serve immediately for optimal freshness and crunch.

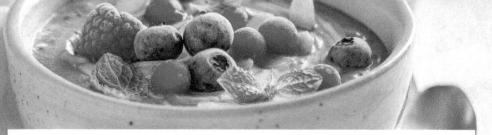

Berry Bliss Smoothie Bowl

INGREDIENTS

- 1 cup frozen mixed berries
- 1/2 banana
- 1/2 cup Greek yogurt
- 1/4 cup almond milk
- 1 tbsp flaxseed
- Toppings: sliced almonds, coconut flakes

PREP. TIME: 10   SERVINGS: 2

DESCRIPTION

A smoothie bowl bursting with antioxidants from mixed berries, with added protein and no added sugars.

DIRECTIONS

1. In a blender, combine frozen berries, banana, Greek yogurt, and almond milk.
2. Blend on high until smooth and creamy.
3. Pour the smoothie mixture into bowls.
4. Top with flaxseed, sliced almonds, and coconut flakes for added texture and nutrients.
5. Serve immediately to enjoy its creamy texture and cold temperature.

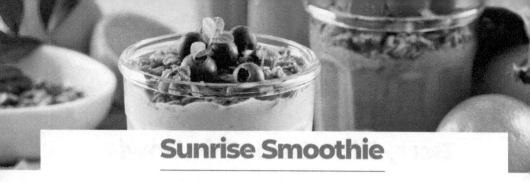

Sunrise Smoothie

INGREDIENTS

- 1 orange, peeled
- 1/2 grapefruit, peeled
- 1 carrot, roughly chopped
- 1 tsp ginger, grated
- 1/2 cup water
- Ice cubes

PREP. TIME: 5   SERVINGS: 2

DESCRIPTION

A bright, citrus-packed smoothie that kick-starts your metabolism and energizes your mornings.

DIRECTIONS

1. Place orange, grapefruit, carrot, and ginger in a blender.
2. Add water and a handful of ice cubes to help blend smoothly.
3. Blend on high until the mixture is smooth.
4. Pour into glasses and serve immediately for a refreshing and energizing start to your day.
5. Optionally, garnish with a slice of orange or a sprig of mint for extra flair.

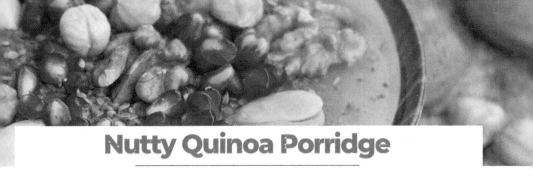

Nutty Quinoa Porridge

INGREDIENTS

- 1 cup quinoa, rinsed
- 2 cups almond milk
- 1/2 tsp cinnamon
- 1 apple, diced
- 2 tbsp walnuts, chopped
- 1 tbsp chia seeds

PREP. TIME:
5

SERVINGS:
3

DESCRIPTION

A warm and satisfying porridge made from quinoa, a complete protein source, topped with nuts and seeds.

DIRECTIONS

1. In a medium saucepan, bring almond milk to a boil.
2. Add quinoa and cinnamon, reduce heat to low and cover. Simmer for 15 minutes or until quinoa is cooked and the mixture thickens.
3. Stir in diced apple during the last 5 minutes of cooking.
4. Once cooked, spoon the porridge into bowls.
5. Top with chopped walnuts and chia seeds for added crunch and nutrients.
6. Serve warm for a hearty, energizing breakfast.

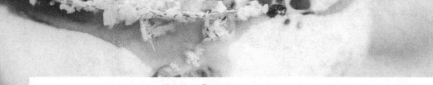

Toasted Coconut Yogurt

INGREDIENTS

- 1 cup Greek yogurt
- 1/2 cup mixed berries
- 1/4 cup granola
- 1/4 cup shredded coconut, toasted
- 1 tbsp honey

PREP. TIME:
10

SERVINGS:
2

DESCRIPTION

A layered parfait with Greek yogurt, toasted coconut, and fresh berries. A perfect balance of protein and fresh flavors.

DIRECTIONS

1. Toast the shredded coconut in a dry skillet over medium heat until golden brown, stirring frequently to prevent burning. Set aside to cool.
2. In serving glasses, layer Greek yogurt at the bottom.
3. Add a layer of mixed berries over the yogurt.
4. Sprinkle granola over the berries, then add another layer of yogurt.
5. Top with toasted coconut and drizzle with honey.
6. Serve immediately or chill in the refrigerator until ready to serve for a cool, refreshing breakfast treat.

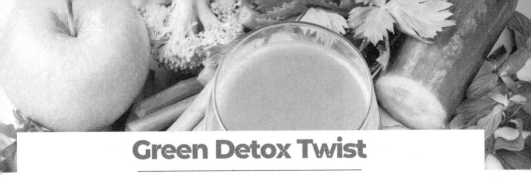

Green Detox Twist

INGREDIENTS

- 1 cup spinach
- 1 cucumber, sliced
- 1 apple, sliced
- 1/2 lemon, juiced
- 1 inch piece of ginger, peeled and sliced

PREP. TIME: 10

SERVINGS: 2

DESCRIPTION

A refreshing green juice blend with spinach, cucumber, and apple, designed to detoxify and energize.

DIRECTIONS

1. Thoroughly wash all vegetables and fruits.
2. In a juicer, combine spinach, cucumber, apple, lemon juice, and ginger.
3. Process until smooth.
4. Pour the juice through a strainer if a smoother texture is desired.
5. Serve the juice immediately to benefit from all the vitamins and enzymes.
6. Optionally, add ice cubes for a refreshing, chilled beverage.

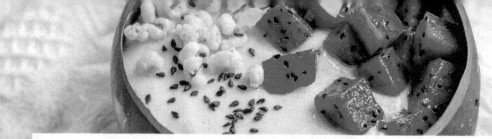

Golden Turmeric Oat Bowl

INGREDIENTS

- 1 cup rolled oats
- 2 cups almond milk
- 1 tsp turmeric powder
- 1 tbsp honey
- 1/2 tsp cinnamon
- 1/4 cup pomegranate seeds
- 1 tbsp almond slivers

PREP. TIME: 10   SERVINGS: 2

DESCRIPTION

Anti-inflammatory oats infused with turmeric and topped with pomegranate seeds, perfect for immune boosting.

DIRECTIONS

1. In a small pot, bring almond milk to a gentle boil.
2. Stir in the oats, turmeric, and cinnamon, reducing heat to a simmer.
3. Cook for 10 minutes, stirring occasionally, until the oats are soft and creamy.
4. Remove from heat and stir in honey for natural sweetness.
5. Serve in bowls, topping each with pomegranate seeds and almond slivers for a crunch and burst of flavor.
6. Enjoy this warm, soothing bowl that kick-starts your metabolism and soothes your body.

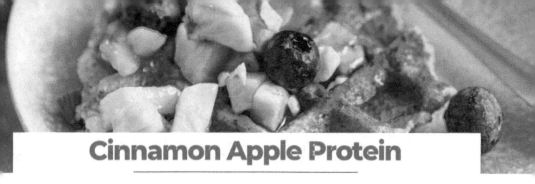

Cinnamon Apple Protein

INGREDIENTS

- 1 cup almond flour
- 2 large eggs
- 1/2 cup Greek yogurt
- 1 tsp cinnamon
- 1 apple, peeled and sliced
- 2 tbsp coconut oil
- 1 tbsp maple syrup

PREP. TIME: 15

SERVINGS: 3

DESCRIPTION

High-protein waffles made with almond flour and topped with sautéed cinnamon apples, perfect for a filling start.

DIRECTIONS

1. Preheat your waffle iron.
2. In a large bowl, mix almond flour, eggs, Greek yogurt, and 1/2 tsp cinnamon to create the batter.
3. Grease the waffle iron with a little coconut oil, then pour in the batter, cooking according to the machine‚Äôs instructions until golden and crispy.
4. Meanwhile, heat the remaining coconut oil in a pan over medium heat and sauté the apple slices with the remaining cinnamon until soft and caramelized.
5. Serve the waffles topped with cinnamon apples and a drizzle of maple syrup.

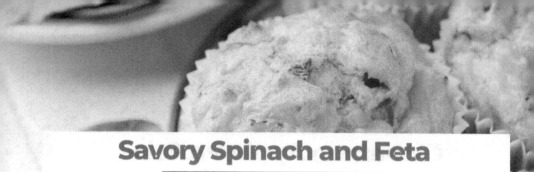

Savory Spinach and Feta

INGREDIENTS

- 2 cups spinach, chopped
- 1 cup almond flour
- 1/2 cup feta cheese, crumbled
- 2 eggs
- 1/4 cup milk
- 1/4 cup olive oil
- 1 tsp baking powder
- Salt and pepper

PREP. TIME: 20 SERVINGS: 6

DESCRIPTION

Savory muffins packed with spinach and feta cheese, offering a perfect blend of protein and greens.

DIRECTIONS

1. Preheat the oven to 350°F (175°C) and grease a muffin tin.
2. In a skillet, sauté spinach until wilted, then set aside to cool.
3. In a bowl, mix almond flour, baking powder, salt, and pepper.
4. In another bowl, whisk eggs, milk, and olive oil.
5. Combine wet and dry ingredients, then fold in the spinach and crumbled feta.
6. Spoon the mixture into the muffin tin and bake for 25 minutes or until the tops are golden and a toothpick comes out clean.
7. Serve warm for a nutrient-rich, savory breakfast option.

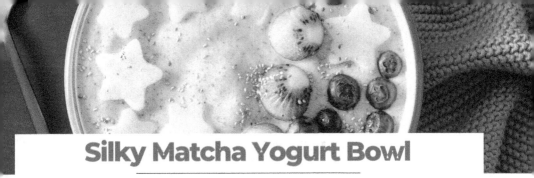

Silky Matcha Yogurt Bowl

INGREDIENTS

- 1 cup Greek yogurt
- 1 tsp matcha powder
- 1 kiwi, sliced
- 1 tbsp pumpkin seeds
- 1 tbsp sunflower seeds
- 1 tsp honey

PREP. TIME: 5

SERVINGS: 2

DESCRIPTION

Energizing matcha mixed with Greek yogurt, topped with kiwi and seeds, for a powerful start to the day.

DIRECTIONS

1. In a bowl, blend the Greek yogurt with matcha powder until smooth.
2. Drizzle honey over the yogurt and stir well to incorporate.
3. Arrange sliced kiwi on top of the yogurt.
4. Sprinkle pumpkin and sunflower seeds for added texture and nutrients.
5. Serve immediately to enjoy the full flavor and benefits of matcha with the creamy texture of yogurt.

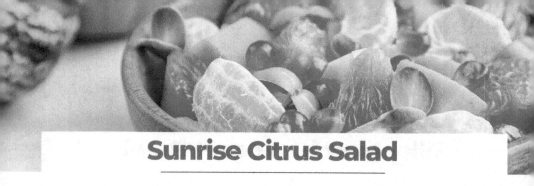

Sunrise Citrus Salad

INGREDIENTS

- 2 oranges, peeled and sectioned
- 1 grapefruit, peeled and sectioned
- 1/2 lime, juiced
- 2 tsp honey
- Fresh mint leaves

PREP. TIME: 10

SERVINGS: 2

DESCRIPTION

Fresh citrus fruits with a hint of mint and a honey-lime dressing, refreshing and perfect for metabolism boosting.

DIRECTIONS

1. In a bowl, combine orange and grapefruit sections.
2. In a small bowl, whisk together lime juice and honey until well combined.
3. Pour the dressing over the citrus fruits and toss gently to coat.
4. Chill the salad in the refrigerator for 10 minutes to blend the flavors.
5. Serve chilled, garnished with fresh mint leaves for an extra refreshing taste.

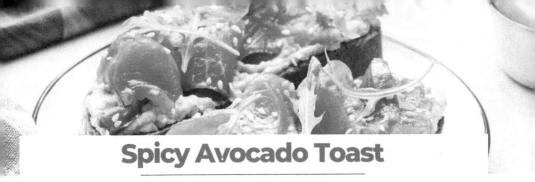

Spicy Avocado Toast

INGREDIENTS

- 2 slices of low-carb bread
- 1 ripe avocado
- 2 eggs
- 1/2 cup fresh salsa
- 1 tbsp olive oil
- Salt and pepper
- 1/2 tsp chili flakes

PREP. TIME: SERVINGS:
5   2

DESCRIPTION

Spicy, heart-healthy avocado toast topped with salsa and poached eggs, for a fiery and nutritious breakfast.

DIRECTIONS

1. Toast the bread slices to your desired crispiness.
2. While the bread is toasting, poach the eggs in simmering water until the whites are set but yolks remain runny, about 3-4 minutes.
3. Mash the avocado with salt, pepper, and chili flakes, then spread evenly on each slice of toast.
4. Top each slice with poached eggs and spoon over fresh salsa.
5. Drizzle with olive oil before serving for a rich, spicy start to your morning.

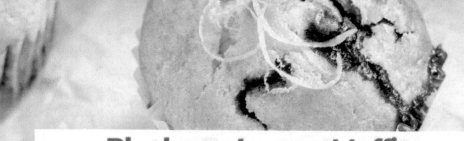

Blueberry Lemon Muffins

INGREDIENTS

- 1 1/2 cups almond flour
- 1/4 cup erythritol (or other keto-friendly sweetener)
- 1 tsp baking powder
- 2 eggs
- 1/4 cup coconut oil, melted
- 1 tsp lemon zest
- 1/2 cup blueberries

PREP. TIME: 15

SERVINGS: 6

DESCRIPTION

Low-carb, keto-friendly muffins bursting with blueberries and a zest of lemon, ideal for a sweet but healthy treat.

DIRECTIONS

1. Preheat the oven to 350°F (175°C) and line a muffin tin with paper liners.
2. In a bowl, combine almond flour, erythritol, and baking powder.
3. In another bowl, whisk together eggs, melted coconut oil, and lemon zest.
4. Mix the wet ingredients into the dry until just combined, then gently fold in blueberries.
5. Divide the batter evenly among the muffin cups.
6. Bake for 20 minutes or until the tops are golden and a toothpick comes out clean.
7. Cool in the tin before serving to enjoy a guilt-free indulgence.

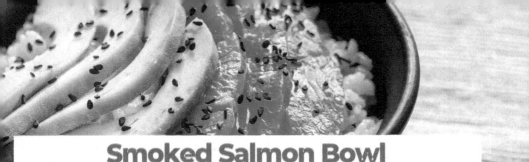

Smoked Salmon Bowl

INGREDIENTS

- 4 oz smoked salmon
- 1 ripe avocado, sliced
- 2 cups arugula
- 1/2 lemon, juiced
- 2 tbsp olive oil
- Salt and pepper
- Capers, for garnish

PREP. TIME: 10   SERVINGS: 2

DESCRIPTION

Omega-rich smoked salmon with avocado and arugula, dressed in a lemon vinaigrette, for a protein-packed breakfast.

DIRECTIONS

1. In a bowl, whisk together lemon juice, olive oil, salt, and pepper to make the dressing.
2. Arrange arugula as the base in two bowls.
3. Top with slices of avocado and smoked salmon.
4. Drizzle the dressing over the salad.
5. Garnish with capers for a burst of flavor.
6. Serve immediately to enjoy a refreshing and satisfying meal.

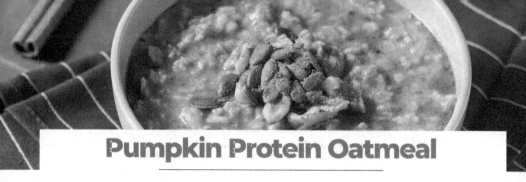

Pumpkin Protein Oatmeal

INGREDIENTS

- 1 cup rolled oats
- 2 cups almond milk
- 1/2 cup pumpkin puree
- 1 scoop vanilla protein powder
- 1 tsp pumpkin spice
- 1 tbsp maple syrup
- Pecans, for topping

PREP. TIME: 5   SERVINGS: 2

DESCRIPTION

Warm, spiced oatmeal packed with protein and fiber, featuring pumpkin puree and spices, for a cozy morning meal.

DIRECTIONS

1. In a pot, bring almond milk to a boil.
2. Add oats and pumpkin spice, then reduce heat to simmer.
3. Stir in pumpkin puree and protein powder, mixing until smooth.
4. Cook for about 10 minutes or until oats are soft.
5. Remove from heat and drizzle with maple syrup.
6. Serve topped with pecans for added crunch and flavor.

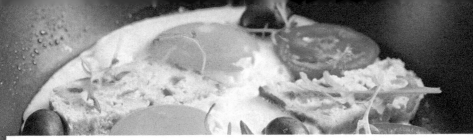

Mediterranean Egg White

INGREDIENTS

- 4 egg whites
- 1/2 cup cherry tomatoes, halved
- 1/4 cup black olives, sliced
- 1/4 cup feta cheese, crumbled
- 1 tbsp olive oil
- Salt and pepper
- Fresh herbs, for garnish

PREP. TIME: 15

SERVINGS: 2

DESCRIPTION

A light and flavorful egg white skillet with tomatoes, olives, and feta, embodying the heart-healthy Mediterranean diet.

DIRECTIONS

1. Heat olive oil in a non-stick skillet over medium heat.
2. Add cherry tomatoes and cook until they start to soften, about 5 minutes.
3. Pour in the egg whites, seasoning with salt and pepper.
4. Cook without stirring for a few minutes until the edges start to set.
5. Sprinkle over olives and feta cheese, then cover and cook until the egg whites are fully set, about 5 minutes.
6. Garnish with fresh herbs before serving to enhance the Mediterranean flavors.

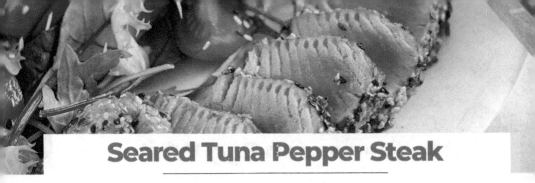

Seared Tuna Pepper Steak

INGREDIENTS

- 2 tuna steaks (6 oz each)
- 1 tbsp cracked black pepper
- Salt
- 1 tbsp olive oil
- 1 orange, juiced
- Mixed herbs (parsley, cilantro)
- Mixed greens

PREP. TIME: 15

SERVINGS: 2

DESCRIPTION

A zesty, low-carb seared tuna steak encrusted with cracked peppercorns, served with a light citrus herb salad.

DIRECTIONS

1. Pat tuna steaks dry and season generously with cracked black pepper and salt.
2. Heat olive oil in a skillet over high heat.
3. Sear the tuna for about 2 minutes on each side or to desired doneness.
4. Whisk together orange juice and chopped herbs for the dressing.
5. Toss mixed greens in the dressing and serve alongside the seared tuna.
6. Garnish with extra herbs and serve immediately.

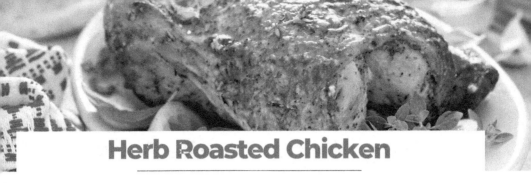

Herb Roasted Chicken

INGREDIENTS

- 1 whole chicken (about 4 lbs)
- 2 lemons, juiced and zested
- 1/4 cup olive oil
- Garlic cloves, minced
- Fresh herbs (rosemary, thyme)
- Salt and pepper

PREP. TIME: 20   SERVINGS: 4

DESCRIPTION

Herb-infused roasted chicken with a tangy lemon glaze, perfect for a comforting yet healthy dinner.

DIRECTIONS

1. Preheat oven to 400°F (200°C).
2. In a bowl, mix lemon juice and zest, olive oil, minced garlic, chopped herbs, salt, and pepper.
3. Rub the mixture all over the chicken, including under the skin.
4. Place chicken in a roasting pan and roast for about 50 minutes or until the juices run clear.
5. Baste occasionally with the pan juices.
6. Let rest for 10 minutes before carving.
7. Serve with a side of steamed vegetables or a green salad.

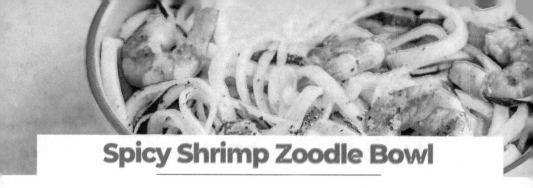

Spicy Shrimp Zoodle Bowl

INGREDIENTS

- 1 lb shrimp, peeled and deveined
- 2 large zucchinis, spiralized
- 1/2 cup tomato sauce
- 1 tsp chili flakes
- 2 cloves garlic, minced
- 1 tbsp olive oil
- Fresh basil

PREP. TIME: 15   SERVINGS: 2

DESCRIPTION

Fresh zucchini noodles tossed with spicy shrimp and a tangy tomato sauce, a light but flavorful dish.

DIRECTIONS

1. Heat olive oil in a large skillet over medium heat.
2. Add minced garlic and chili flakes, sauté for 1 minute.
3. Add shrimp and cook until pink, about 2-3 minutes per side.
4. Toss in spiralized zucchini and tomato sauce, cook for about 3-5 minutes until zoodles are tender but still firm.
5. Garnish with fresh basil before serving.
6. Serve hot for a light and spicy meal.

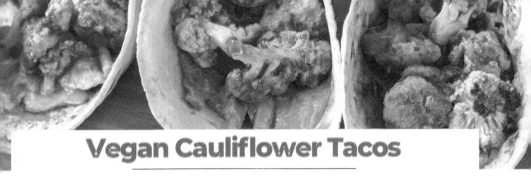

Vegan Cauliflower Tacos

INGREDIENTS

- 1 head cauliflower, cut into florets
- 1 tbsp smoked paprika
- 2 avocados
- 1 lime, juiced
- Fresh cilantro
- Corn tortillas
- Salt and olive oil

PREP. TIME: 10

SERVINGS: 4

DESCRIPTION

Smoky roasted cauliflower tacos topped with a vibrant avocado cilantro sauce, a vegan delight.

DIRECTIONS

1. Preheat oven to 425°F (220°C).
2. Toss cauliflower florets with olive oil, smoked paprika, and salt.
3. Roast in the oven for 15 minutes until tender and charred at the edges.
4. Blend avocados, lime juice, and cilantro to make a creamy sauce.
5. Warm tortillas in a skillet.
6. Assemble tacos with roasted cauliflower and drizzle with avocado cilantro sauce.
7. Serve immediately, garnished with extra cilantro.

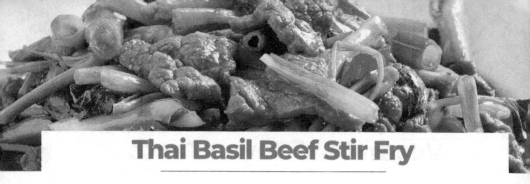

Thai Basil Beef Stir Fry

INGREDIENTS

- 1/2 lb beef sirloin, thinly sliced
- 1 bunch Thai basil leaves
- 2 cloves garlic, minced
- 2 tbsp soy sauce (or tamari for gluten-free)
- 1 tbsp fish sauce
- 1 tbsp oil

PREP. TIME: 10

SERVINGS: 2

DESCRIPTION

Quick and fiery Thai basil beef, perfect for a spicy and satisfying low-carb dinner.

DIRECTIONS

1. Heat oil in a wok or large skillet over high heat.
2. Add minced garlic and sauté until fragrant, about 30 seconds.
3. Add beef and stir-fry until it starts to brown, about 2-3 minutes.
4. Stir in soy sauce and fish sauce.
5. Add Thai basil leaves and cook until wilted, about 1-2 minutes.
6. Serve hot over cauliflower rice or alongside steamed vegetables for a complete meal.

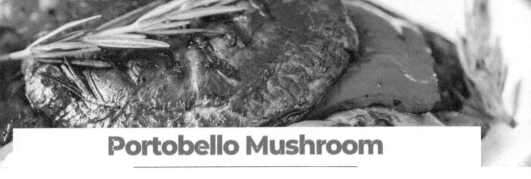

Portobello Mushroom

INGREDIENTS

- 4 large portobello mush-rooms, stems removed
- 1/4 cup balsamic vinegar
- 2 cloves garlic, minced
- 1/4 cup olive oil
- Fresh thyme
- Salt and pepper

PREP. TIME: 15   SERVINGS: 4

DESCRIPTION

Juicy portobello steaks with a balsamic garlic marinade, a hearty vege-tarian option that satisfies.

DIRECTIONS

1. In a small bowl, whisk together balsamic vinegar, olive oil, minced garlic, thyme, salt, and pepper.
2. Place mushroom caps in a dish and pour marinade over them. Let marinate for at least 15 minutes.
3. Preheat grill to medium-high heat.
4. Grill mushrooms for about 5 minutes on each side or until tender and grill marks appear.
5. Serve with a side salad or roasted vegetables.
6. Drizzle with extra marinade from the dish before serving.

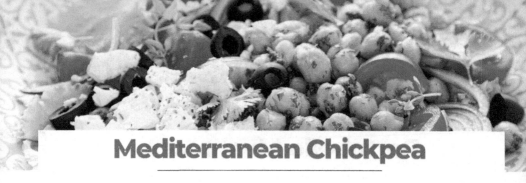

Mediterranean Chickpea

INGREDIENTS

- 2 cans chickpeas, drained and rinsed
- 1/2 cup kalamata olives, pitted
- 1/2 cup sun-dried tomatoes, chopped
- 1/4 cup feta cheese, crumbled
- 1 lemon, juiced
- 1/4 cup olive oil
- Fresh parsley

PREP. TIME:
20

SERVINGS:
4

DESCRIPTION

A refreshing bowl of chickpeas, kalamata olives, feta, and sun-dried tomatoes, dressed in a lemony vinaigrette.

DIRECTIONS

1. In a large bowl, combine chickpeas, olives, sun-dried tomatoes, and crumbled feta.
2. In a small bowl, whisk together lemon juice, olive oil, and a pinch of salt.
3. Pour dressing over the chickpea mixture and toss to coat evenly.
4. Let the salad sit for about 10 minutes to allow flavors to meld.
5. Garnish with chopped parsley before serving.
6. Serve chilled or at room temperature as a light and nutritious main dish.

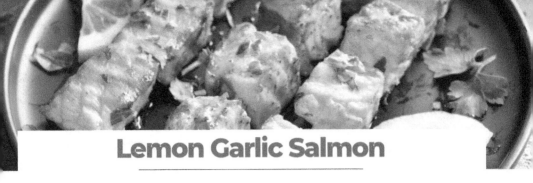

Lemon Garlic Salmon

INGREDIENTS

- 1 lb salmon fillet, cut into cubes
- 2 lemons, juiced and zested
- 3 cloves garlic, minced
- 2 tbsp olive oil
- Salt and pepper
- Wooden or metal skewers

PREP. TIME: 20   SERVINGS: 4

DESCRIPTION

Skewered salmon chunks marinated in lemon and garlic, grilled to perfection for a light meal.

DIRECTIONS

1. In a bowl, combine lemon juice and zest, minced garlic, olive oil, salt, and pepper.
2. Add salmon cubes to the marinade and let sit for at least 30 minutes in the refrigerator.
3. Preheat grill to medium-high heat.
4. Thread marinated salmon onto skewers.
5. Grill for about 3-4 minutes per side or until salmon is cooked through and opaque.
6. Serve hot, garnished with additional lemon slices or fresh herbs.

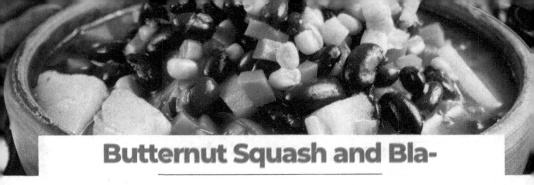

Butternut Squash and Bla-

INGREDIENTS

- 1 butternut squash, peeled and cubed
- 2 cans black beans, drained
- 1 onion, chopped
- 2 cloves garlic, minced
- 1 can diced tomatoes
- 1 tbsp chili powder
- 1 tsp cumin
- Salt and pepper
- 1/4 cup olive oil

PREP. TIME:
20

SERVINGS:
6

DESCRIPTION

A hearty and healthy chili made with butternut squash and black beans, spiced to comfort any palate.

DIRECTIONS

1. Heat olive oil in a large pot over medium heat.
2. Add chopped onion and garlic, sauté until translucent.
3. Stir in butternut squash, diced tomatoes, chili powder, and cumin.
4. Add black beans and enough water to cover all ingredients.
5. Bring to a boil, then reduce heat and simmer for about 30 minutes, or until the squash is tender.
6. Season with salt and pepper to taste.
7. Serve hot, garnished with fresh cilantro or sour cream if desired.

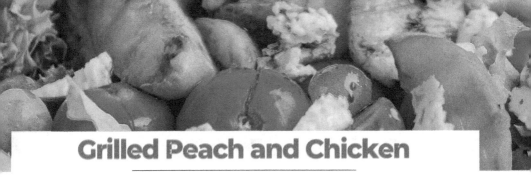

Grilled Peach and Chicken

INGREDIENTS

- 2 peaches, halved and pitted
- 1 lb chicken breasts
- Mixed salad greens
- 1/4 cup honey
- 2 tbsp mustard
- 1/4 cup olive oil
- Salt and pepper

PREP. TIME:
15

SERVINGS:
4

DESCRIPTION

A sweet and savory salad with grilled peaches and chicken, topped with a honey mustard dressing.

DIRECTIONS

1. Season chicken breasts with salt and pepper.
2. Grill chicken on medium-high until cooked through, about 5-6 minutes per side.
3. Grill peaches cut-side down until charred, about 2-3 minutes.
4. Slice chicken and peaches.
5. In a bowl, whisk together honey, mustard, and olive oil to make the dressing.
6. Toss salad greens in half the dressing.
7. Arrange greens on plates, top with chicken and peach slices.
8. Drizzle remaining dressing over the top.
9. Serve immediately.

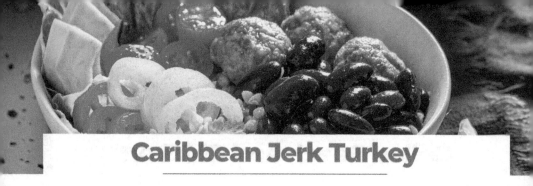

Caribbean Jerk Turkey

INGREDIENTS

- 1 lb ground turkey
- 2 tbsp jerk seasoning
- 1 mango, diced
- 1/2 red bell pepper, diced
- 1/4 cup red onion, diced
- 1 lime, juiced
- 2 cups cauliflower rice

PREP. TIME:
20

SERVINGS:
4

DESCRIPTION

Spicy jerk-seasoned turkey served over a bed of cauliflower rice, paired with mango salsa for a tropical twist.

DIRECTIONS

1. Season ground turkey with jerk seasoning and brown in a skillet over medium heat until cooked through.
2. Prepare the mango salsa by combining diced mango, red bell pepper, red onion, and lime juice in a bowl.
3. Sauté cauliflower rice in a separate pan until heated through and slightly crispy.
4. Serve the cooked turkey over the cauliflower rice.
5. Top with fresh mango salsa.
6. Garnish with cilantro and a lime wedge for added flavor and presentation.

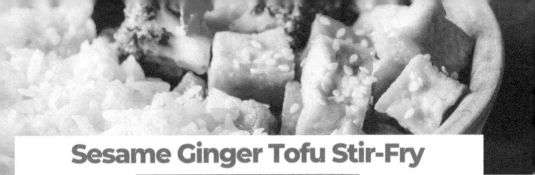

Sesame Ginger Tofu Stir-Fry

INGREDIENTS

- 1 block firm tofu, cubed
- 2 tbsp sesame oil
- 2 cups mixed vegetables (carrots, bell peppers, broccoli)
- 2 tbsp soy sauce
- 1 tbsp fresh ginger, grated
- 1 tbsp sesame seeds

PREP. TIME: 15

SERVINGS: 2

DESCRIPTION

Crisp tofu stir-fried with a medley of vegetables and a savory sesame ginger sauce, ideal for a vegan feast.

DIRECTIONS

1. Press tofu to remove excess water, then cube.
2. Heat sesame oil in a large skillet over medium-high heat.
3. Add tofu and cook until golden on all sides.
4. Add vegetables and stir-fry until just tender.
5. Mix in soy sauce and grated ginger, cooking for an additional minute.
6. Sprinkle with sesame seeds before serving.
7. Serve hot, garnished with green onions or additional sesame seeds if desired.

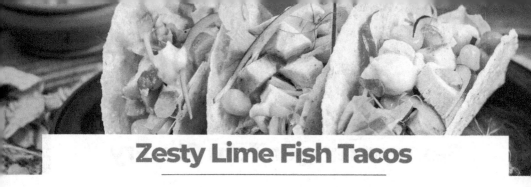

Zesty Lime Fish Tacos

INGREDIENTS

- 1 lb white fish (like tilapia)
- 2 limes, juiced
- 1 tsp chili powder
- 8 small corn tortillas
- 1 cup red cabbage, shredded
- 1 avocado, sliced
- Fresh cilantro

PREP. TIME: 10   SERVINGS: 4

DESCRIPTION

Light and flavorful fish tacos with a zesty lime infusion, topped with a fresh cabbage slaw for a crunchy texture.

DIRECTIONS

1. Marinate fish with lime juice and chili powder for 10 minutes.
2. Cook fish in a skillet over medium heat until flaky and cooked through, about 3-4 minutes per side.
3. Warm tortillas in a dry skillet or on the grill.
4. Assemble tacos with fish, shredded cabbage, sliced avocado, and fresh cilantro.
5. Serve with extra lime wedges and enjoy a burst of freshness in every bite.

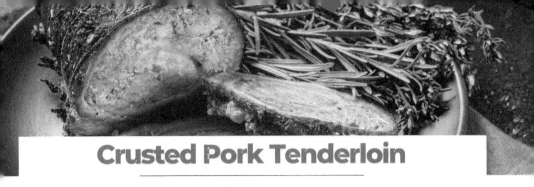

Crusted Pork Tenderloin

INGREDIENTS

- 1 pork tenderloin (about 1 lb)
- 1 tbsp olive oil
- 1 tbsp rosemary, minced
- 1 tbsp thyme, minced
- 1 tbsp garlic, minced
- Salt and pepper

PREP. TIME: 15   SERVINGS: 4

DESCRIPTION

A juicy pork tenderloin encrusted with fragrant herbs, roasted to perfection for a tender and savory centerpiece.

DIRECTIONS

1. Preheat oven to 375°F (190°C).
2. Rub pork with olive oil, then coat with minced herbs, garlic, salt, and pepper.
3. Roast in the oven until the internal temperature reaches 145°F (63°C), about 25 minutes.
4. Let rest for 5 minutes before slicing.
5. Serve with a side of roasted vegetables or a fresh salad.

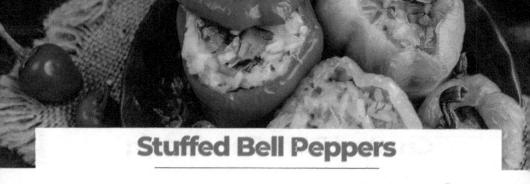

Stuffed Bell Peppers

INGREDIENTS

- 4 bell peppers, halved and seeded
- 1 cup quinoa, cooked
- 1 can black beans, rinsed and drained
- 1 cup corn
- 1/2 cup tomato sauce
- 1 tsp cumin
- 1 tsp chili powder
- 1/2 cup shredded cheese (optional)

PREP. TIME: 20   SERVINGS: 4

DESCRIPTION

Colorful bell peppers stuffed with a savory mixture of quinoa, black beans, corn, and spices, baked to perfection.

DIRECTIONS

1. Preheat oven to 350°F (175°C).
2. In a bowl, mix cooked quinoa, black beans, corn, tomato sauce, cumin, and chili powder.
3. Stuff the bell pepper halves with the quinoa mixture.
4. Top with shredded cheese, if using.
5. Bake for 30 minutes, or until the peppers are tender and the filling is heated through.
6. Garnish with fresh cilantro or sour cream before serving.

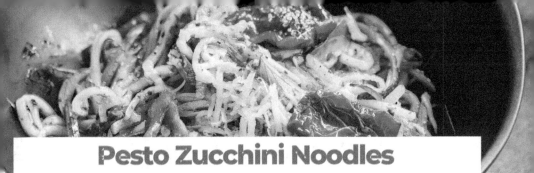

Pesto Zucchini Noodles

INGREDIENTS

- 2 zucchinis, spiralized
- 1/2 cup basil leaves
- 1/4 cup pine nuts
- 2 cloves garlic
- 1/4 cup olive oil
- 1/4 cup grated Parmesan cheese
- Salt and pepper

PREP. TIME:
10

SERVINGS:
2

DESCRIPTION

Spiralized zucchini noo-
dles tossed in a home-
made pesto sauce, a light
and flavorful dish that's
both nutritious and satisfying.

DIRECTIONS

1. In a food processor, combine basil leaves, pine nuts, garlic, and olive oil to create the pesto.
2. Blend until smooth, then stir in grated Parmesan, salt, and pepper to taste.
3. Toss spiralized zucchini with the pesto until well coated.
4. Serve immediately, topped with additional Parmesan cheese and a sprinkle of red pepper flakes for a spicy kick.

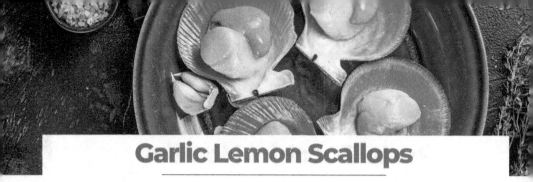

Garlic Lemon Scallops

INGREDIENTS

- 1 lb scallops
- 2 tbsp butter
- 2 cloves garlic, minced
- 1 lemon, juiced and zested
- Fresh parsley
- Salt and pepper

PREP. TIME:
10

SERVINGS:
2

DESCRIPTION

Seared scallops with a garlic lemon butter sauce, a luxurious yet simple dish that brings the ocean's freshness to your plate.

DIRECTIONS

1. Pat scallops dry and season with salt and pepper.
2. Heat butter in a skillet over medium-high heat.
3. Add scallops, cooking without moving until golden on one side, about 2-3 minutes.
4. Flip scallops, add garlic, and cook for another 2 minutes.
5. Pour in lemon juice and zest, then garnish with parsley before serving.
6. Serve hot with a side of steamed asparagus or over a bed of fresh greens.

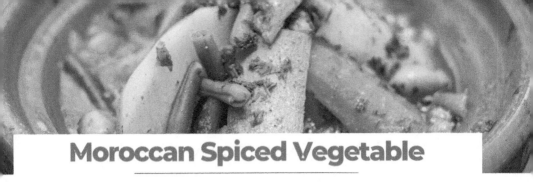

Moroccan Spiced Vegetable

INGREDIENTS

- 1 sweet potato, cubed
- 2 carrots, sliced
- 1 zucchini, sliced
- 1 bell pepper, chopped
- 1 onion, chopped
- 2 cloves garlic, minced
- 1 tsp cumin
- 1 tsp coriander
- 1/2 tsp cinnamon
- 1 can diced tomatoes
- 1/4 cup dried apricots, chopped

PREP. TIME: 20
SERVINGS: 4

DESCRIPTION

Aromatic spices and a medley of vegetables slow-cooked in a traditional tagine, offering a taste of North Africa.

DIRECTIONS

1. Heat a large pot or tagine over medium heat.
2. Add olive oil and onion, sauté until translucent.
3. Stir in garlic, spices, and vegetables, cooking for a few minutes to release flavors.
4. Add diced tomatoes and dried apricots, bring to a simmer.
5. Cover and cook on low heat for 40 minutes, or until vegetables are tender.
6. Garnish with fresh cilantro and serve with couscous or flatbread.

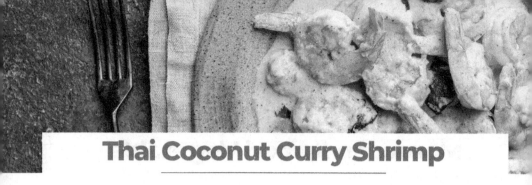

Thai Coconut Curry Shrimp

INGREDIENTS

- 1 lb shrimp, peeled and deveined
- 1 can coconut milk
- 1 tbsp Thai curry paste
- 1 bell pepper, sliced
- 1 onion, sliced
- 1 tbsp fish sauce
- Fresh basil
- 1 lime, juiced

PREP. TIME: 15

SERVINGS: 4

DESCRIPTION

Creamy coconut curry with shrimp, infused with Thai spices and served over jasmine rice for a comforting meal.

DIRECTIONS

1. Heat a skillet over medium heat and sauté onion and bell pepper until soft.
2. Stir in curry paste and cook for 1 minute.
3. Add coconut milk and fish sauce, bringing to a simmer.
4. Add shrimp and cook until they turn pink, about 3-5 minutes.
5. Stir in lime juice and garnish with fresh basil.
6. Serve over steamed jasmine rice, garnished with extra basil leaves.

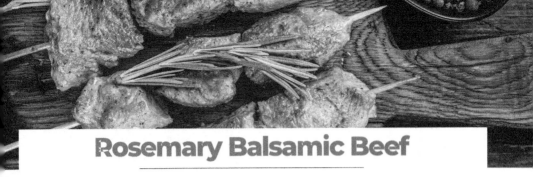

Rosemary Balsamic Beef

INGREDIENTS

- 1 lb beef sirloin, cut into cubes
- 1/4 cup balsamic vinegar
- 1/4 cup olive oil
- 2 tbsp rosemary, chopped
- 2 cloves garlic, minced
- Salt and pepper

PREP. TIME: 20   SERVINGS: 4

DESCRIPTION

Grilled beef skewers marinated in a rosemary balsamic reduction, offering a robust flavor that's both tender and tantalizing.

DIRECTIONS

1. In a bowl, whisk together balsamic vinegar, olive oil, rosemary, garlic, salt, and pepper.
2. Marinate beef cubes in the mixture for at least 30 minutes.
3. Thread beef onto skewers.
4. Preheat grill to medium-high heat.
5. Grill skewers, turning occasionally, until cooked to desired doneness, about 8-10 minutes.
6. Serve hot, paired with a fresh garden salad or grilled vegetables.
7. Drizzle with remaining marinade for added flavor.

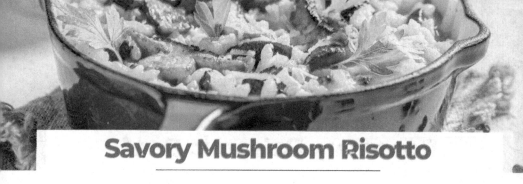

Savory Mushroom Risotto

INGREDIENTS

- 1 cup arborio rice
- 3 cups vegetable broth, heated
- 1 cup mixed mushrooms, sliced
- 1/2 cup white wine
- 1 onion, finely chopped
- 2 cloves garlic, minced
- 1/4 cup Parmesan cheese, grated
- 2 tbsp olive oil
- Fresh parsley, chopped
- Salt and pepper

PREP. TIME: 20   SERVINGS: 4

DESCRIPTION

A creamy and aromatic risotto made with assorted mushrooms and a hint of white wine, perfect for a comforting, low-fat dinner.

DIRECTIONS

1. In a large pan, heat olive oil over medium heat.
2. Add onions and garlic, sauté until translucent.
3. Stir in mushrooms and cook until they begin to release their juices.
4. Add arborio rice, stir to coat with oil and toast lightly.
5. Pour in white wine, let simmer until mostly absorbed.
6. Add warm broth one ladle at a time, allowing each addition to be absorbed before adding the next.
7. Continue until rice is creamy and al dente.
8. Stir in Parmesan cheese and season with salt and pepper.
9. Garnish with fresh parsley and serve immediately.

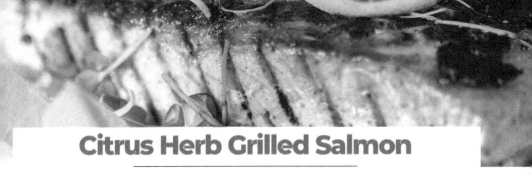

Citrus Herb Grilled Salmon

INGREDIENTS

- 4 salmon fillets
- 2 lemons, juiced and zested
- 1 orange, juiced and zested
- 2 tbsp olive oil
- 1 tbsp fresh dill, chopped
- 1 tbsp fresh parsley, chopped
- Salt and pepper
- 1 lb green beans

PREP. TIME:
15

SERVINGS:
4

DESCRIPTION

Grilled salmon fillets marinated in a citrus herb mixture, served with a side of steamed green beans for a refreshing meal.

DIRECTIONS

1. In a bowl, mix lemon juice, orange juice, olive oil, dill, parsley, salt, and pepper.
2. Marinate the salmon fillets in the citrus herb mixture for at least 30 minutes.
3. Preheat grill to medium-high heat.
4. Grill salmon for about 5 minutes on each side, depending on thickness, until cooked through.
5. Simultaneously, steam the green beans until tender.
6. Serve the grilled salmon with a side of steamed green beans, garnished with additional herbs or lemon slices.

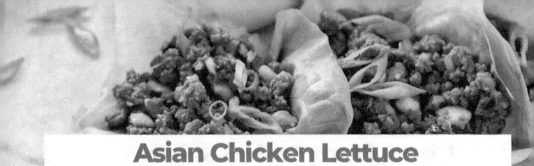

Asian Chicken Lettuce

INGREDIENTS

- 1 lb ground chicken
- 1 can water chestnuts, finely chopped
- 1/2 onion, chopped
- 2 cloves garlic, minced
- 1/4 cup hoisin sauce
- 2 tbsp soy sauce
- 1 tbsp sesame oil
- 1 head iceberg lettuce, separated into leaves
- Fresh cilantro, for garnish

PREP. TIME: 15

SERVINGS: 4

DESCRIPTION

Crunchy lettuce wraps filled with savory chicken, water chestnuts, and a sweet hoisin sauce, ideal for a light and healthy meal.

DIRECTIONS

1. Heat sesame oil in a skillet over medium heat.
2. Add onion and garlic, sauté until softened.
3. Add ground chicken, cook until browned and crumbled.
4. Stir in water chestnuts, hoisin sauce, and soy sauce; cook until heated through.
5. Spoon chicken mixture into lettuce leaves.
6. Garnish with fresh cilantro and serve immediately.

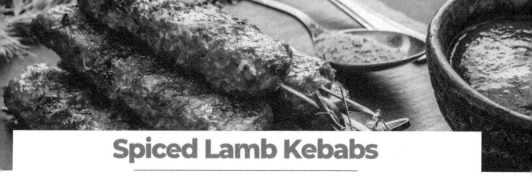

Spiced Lamb Kebabs

INGREDIENTS

- 1 lb lamb, cut into cubes
- 2 tbsp olive oil
- 1 tsp cumin
- 1 tsp coriander
- 1/2 tsp cinnamon
- 1/2 tsp allspice
- Salt and pepper
- 1 cucumber, grated
- 1 cup Greek yogurt
- 1 lemon, juiced
- Fresh mint, chopped

PREP. TIME: 25 SERVINGS: 4

DESCRIPTION

Flavorful lamb kebabs marinated in a blend of Middle Eastern spices, grilled to perfection and served with yogurt cucumber sauce.

DIRECTIONS

1. In a bowl, mix olive oil, cumin, coriander, cinnamon, allspice, salt, and pepper.
2. Add lamb cubes to the marinade and let sit for at least 1 hour in the refrigerator.
3. Preheat the grill to medium-high heat.
4. Thread lamb onto skewers.
5. Grill for about 6-8 minutes, turning occasionally, until cooked to desired doneness.
6. For the sauce, combine Greek yogurt, grated cucumber, lemon juice, and mint in a bowl.
7. Serve lamb kebabs with cucumber yogurt sauce on the side.

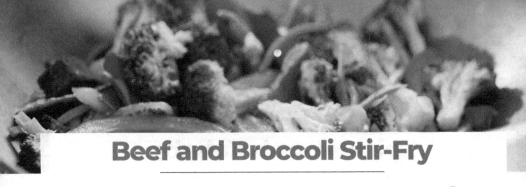

Beef and Broccoli Stir-Fry

INGREDIENTS

- 1 lb beef sirloin, thinly sliced
- 2 cups broccoli florets
- 1/2 onion, sliced
- 2 cloves garlic, minced
- 1/4 cup soy sauce
- 2 tbsp sesame oil
- 1 tbsp cornstarch
- 1/4 cup water

PREP. TIME: 10   SERVINGS: 4

DESCRIPTION

A classic beef and broccoli stir-fry with a soy sauce glaze, offering a high-protein and low-carb dinner option.

DIRECTIONS

1. In a small bowl, mix cornstarch and water to create a slurry.
2. Heat sesame oil in a large skillet over medium-high heat.
3. Add garlic and onion, sauté until soft.
4. Add beef and stir-fry until it starts to brown.
5. Add broccoli and continue to cook until vegetables are tender.
6. Pour soy sauce and cornstarch slurry over the beef and broccoli, stirring constantly until the sauce thickens.
7. Serve immediately, ideal with a side of cauliflower rice.

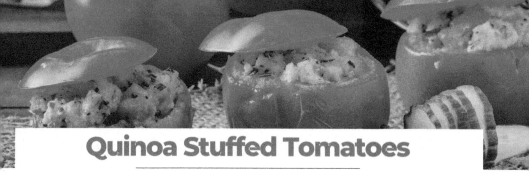

Quinoa Stuffed Tomatoes

INGREDIENTS

- 4 large tomatoes
- 1 cup quinoa, cooked
- 1 cup spinach, chopped
- 1/2 cup feta cheese, crumbled
- 2 cloves garlic, minced
- Salt and pepper
- 2 tbsp olive oil
- Fresh basil, for garnish

PREP. TIME: 15   SERVINGS: 4

DESCRIPTION

Baked tomatoes stuffed with a flavorful quinoa mixture, featuring spinach and feta, for a nutritious vegetarian main dish.

DIRECTIONS

1. Preheat oven to 375°F (190°C).
2. Cut off the tops of the tomatoes and scoop out the insides.
3. In a bowl, mix cooked quinoa, spinach, feta, garlic, salt, and pepper.
4. Stuff the tomatoes with the quinoa mixture.
5. Place stuffed tomatoes in a baking dish, drizzle with olive oil.
6. Bake for 20 minutes, until the tomatoes are tender and the filling is heated through.
7. Garnish with fresh basil and serve hot.

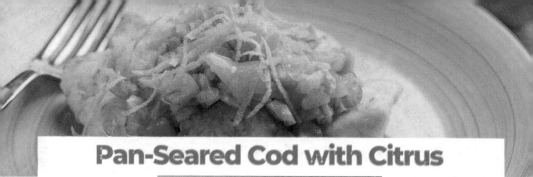

Pan-Seared Cod with Citrus

INGREDIENTS

- 4 cod fillets
- 2 oranges, segmented
- 1 grapefruit, segmented
- 1 lime, juiced
- 1/4 red onion, finely chopped
- 1 jalape√±o, finely chopped
- Salt and pepper
- 2 tbsp olive oil

PREP. TIME: 15   SERVINGS: 4

DESCRIPTION

Lightly seared cod fillets topped with a fresh citrus salsa for a light, refreshing main course.

DIRECTIONS

1. Season cod fillets with salt and pepper.
2. Heat olive oil in a non-stick skillet over medium heat.
3. Place cod in the skillet, cook for about 6 minutes per side or until opaque and flaky.
4. In a bowl, mix orange and grapefruit segments, lime juice, red onion, and jalape√±o to make the salsa.
5. Top each cod fillet with a generous amount of citrus salsa.
6. Serve immediately, offering a zesty and nutritious dish.

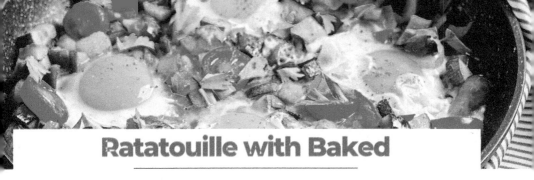

Ratatouille with Baked

INGREDIENTS

- 1 eggplant, sliced
- 2 zucchinis, sliced
- 1 bell pepper, chopped
- 1 onion, chopped
- 3 tomatoes, sliced
- 4 eggs
- 2 tbsp olive oil
- Salt and pepper
- Fresh thyme
- 1 clove garlic, minced

PREP. TIME: 20

SERVINGS: 4

DESCRIPTION

Classic French ratatouille with eggs baked right into the vegetable medley, perfect for a hearty yet healthy meal.

DIRECTIONS

1. Preheat oven to 375°F (190°C).
2. In a large baking dish, layer sliced eggplant, zucchini, bell pepper, onion, and tomatoes.
3. Drizzle with olive oil and sprinkle with salt, pepper, minced garlic, and thyme.
4. Bake for 30 minutes, until vegetables are tender.
5. Make four wells in the ratatouille, crack an egg into each.
6. Return to oven and bake until eggs are set, about 10 minutes.
7. Serve hot, garnished with additional fresh herbs.

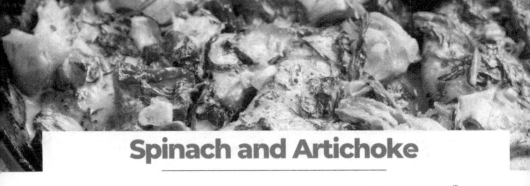

Spinach and Artichoke

INGREDIENTS

- 4 chicken breasts
- 1 can artichoke hearts, drained and chopped
- 1 cup spinach, chopped
- 1/2 cup cream cheese
- 1/4 cup grated Parmesan cheese
- Salt and pepper
- 2 tbsp olive oil

PREP. TIME: 15

SERVINGS: 4

DESCRIPTION

Juicy chicken breasts topped with a creamy spinach and artichoke topping, baked to golden perfection.

DIRECTIONS

1. Preheat oven to 375°F (190°C).
2. Season chicken breasts with salt and pepper.
3. Heat olive oil in a skillet over medium-high heat, sear chicken on both sides until golden.
4. In a bowl, mix cream cheese, chopped artichokes, spinach, and Parmesan.
5. Place seared chicken in a baking dish, top with spinach artichoke mixture.
6. Bake for 25 minutes or until chicken is cooked through and topping is bubbly.
7. Serve hot, garnished with extra Parmesan or fresh herbs.

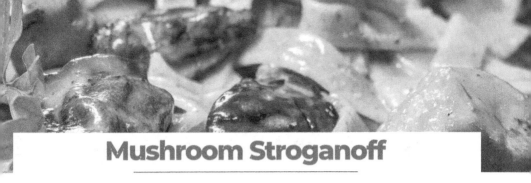

Mushroom Stroganoff

INGREDIENTS

- 1 lb mushrooms, sliced
- 1 onion, chopped
- 2 cloves garlic, minced
- 1 cup vegetable broth
- 1 cup coconut cream
- 2 tbsp soy sauce
- 1 tbsp olive oil
- Fresh parsley, for garnish
- Salt and pepper

PREP. TIME: 15

SERVINGS: 4

DESCRIPTION

A creamy and comforting vegan stroganoff made with sautéed mushrooms and a rich coconut cream sauce.

DIRECTIONS

1. Heat olive oil in a large skillet over medium heat.
2. Add onions and garlic, cook until softened.
3. Add mushrooms, sauté until browned and released their juices.
4. Stir in soy sauce and vegetable broth, bring to a simmer.
5. Add coconut cream, reduce heat, and simmer for about 10 minutes until the sauce thickens.
6. Season with salt and pepper to taste.
7. Serve hot over egg noodles or rice, garnished with fresh parsley.

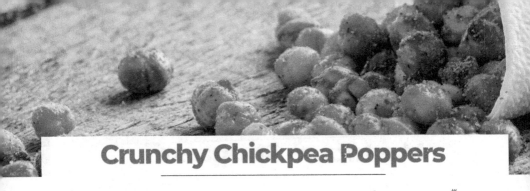

Crunchy Chickpea Poppers

INGREDIENTS

- 2 cans chickpeas, drained and rinsed
- 1 tbsp olive oil
- 1 tsp paprika
- 1/2 tsp cumin
- Salt and pepper

PREP. TIME:
10

SERVINGS:
4

DESCRIPTION

Oven-roasted chickpeas seasoned with a spicy blend, perfect for a crunchy, protein-packed snack.

DIRECTIONS

1. Preheat oven to 400°F (200°C).
2. Pat chickpeas dry with paper towels.
3. Toss chickpeas with olive oil, paprika, cumin, salt, and pepper.
4. Spread on a baking sheet in a single layer.
5. Bake for 30 minutes, stirring occasionally, until crispy.
6. Let cool before serving.

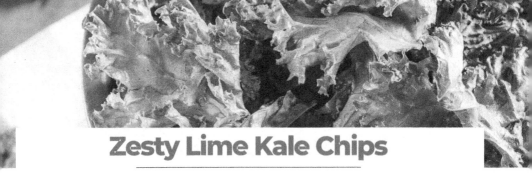

Zesty Lime Kale Chips

INGREDIENTS

- 1 bunch kale, stems removed and leaves torn
- 2 tbsp olive oil
- 1 lime, zested and juiced
- Salt

PREP. TIME:
5

SERVINGS:
2

DESCRIPTION

Crispy kale chips with a tangy lime twist, a low-calorie snack that satisfies the craving for something crunchy.

DIRECTIONS

1. Preheat oven to 300°F (150°C).
2. Massage kale with olive oil, lime juice, and salt.
3. Lay kale pieces on a baking sheet without overlapping.
4. Bake for 15 minutes, or until crisp.
5. Sprinkle with lime zest before serving.
6. Enjoy as a light, crispy snack.

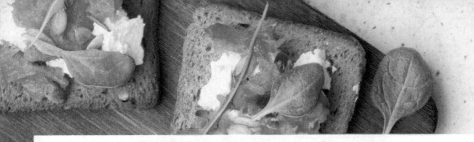

Sweet Potato Toasts

INGREDIENTS

- 2 large sweet potatoes, sliced lengthwise
- 1 avocado, mashed
- 1/2 tsp chili flakes
- Salt and pepper
- Olive oil

PREP. TIME:
5

SERVINGS:
4

DESCRIPTION

Slices of sweet potato toasted and topped with avocado and spices, offering a gluten-free and nutritious alternative.

DIRECTIONS

1. Preheat your toaster or oven to 400°F (200°C).
2. Brush sweet potato slices with olive oil and season with salt and pepper.
3. Toast in batches until tender and edges are crispy, about 15 minutes in the oven.
4. Top each slice with mashed avocado.
5. Sprinkle with chili flakes.
6. Serve immediately as a vibrant, healthy snack.

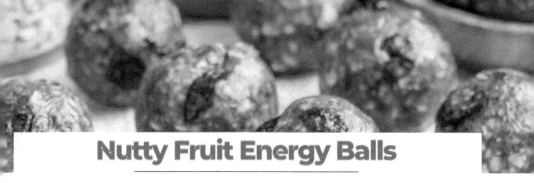

Nutty Fruit Energy Balls

INGREDIENTS

- 1 cup rolled oats
- 1/2 cup mixed nuts, chopped
- 1/2 cup dried cranberries
- 1/2 cup peanut butter
- 1/4 cup honey

PREP. TIME: 15

SERVINGS: 12

DESCRIPTION

No-bake energy balls packed with oats, nuts, and dried fruits, perfect for a quick energy boost.

DIRECTIONS

1. In a large bowl, combine all ingredients until well mixed.
2. Roll the mixture into small balls, about the size of a walnut.
3. Place on a baking sheet lined with parchment paper.
4. Refrigerate for at least 1 hour to set.
5. Enjoy as a grab-and-go snack.

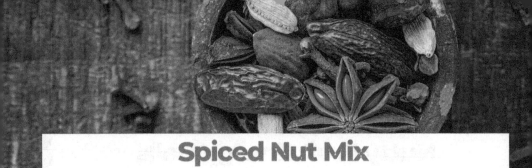

Spiced Nut Mix

INGREDIENTS

- 2 cups mixed nuts (almonds, walnuts, pecans)
- 1 tbsp olive oil
- 1 tsp smoked paprika
- 1/2 tsp garlic powder
- 1/2 tsp salt

PREP. TIME:
5

SERVINGS:
4

DESCRIPTION

A savory mix of roasted nuts seasoned with spices, a perfect healthy snack for any time of day.

DIRECTIONS

1. Preheat oven to 350°F (175°C).
2. In a bowl, toss nuts with olive oil, smoked paprika, garlic powder, and salt.
3. Spread nuts on a baking sheet in a single layer.
4. Roast for 10 minutes, stirring once.
5. Cool before serving.

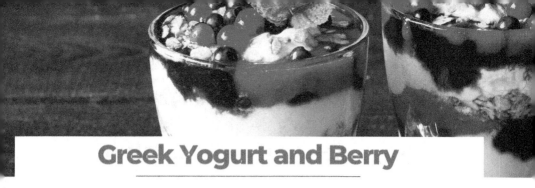

Greek Yogurt and Berry

INGREDIENTS

- 1 cup Greek yogurt
- 1/2 cup granola
- 1/2 cup mixed berries
(blueberries, strawberries)
- 1 tbsp honey

PREP. TIME: 10   SERVINGS: 2

DESCRIPTION

Layers of creamy Greek yogurt, fresh berries, and granola, making it a delicious and filling snack or breakfast option.

DIRECTIONS

1. In two glasses, layer Greek yogurt, granola, and berries.
2. Repeat the layers until all ingredients are used up.
3. Drizzle honey over the top layer.
4. Serve immediately or refrigerate until ready to enjoy.

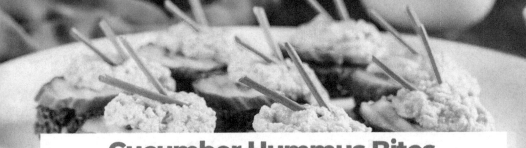

Cucumber Hummus Bites

INGREDIENTS

- 1 cucumber, sliced
- 1 cup hummus
- 1/2 cup cherry tomatoes, halved
- Fresh dill for garnish

PREP. TIME:
10

SERVINGS:
4

DESCRIPTION

Fresh cucumber slices topped with creamy hummus and cherry tomatoes, a refreshing and healthy snack.

DIRECTIONS

1. Arrange cucumber slices on a platter.
2. Top each slice with a spoonful of hummus.
3. Add a cherry tomato half on top.
4. Garnish with dill.
5. Serve as a cool and crisp snack.

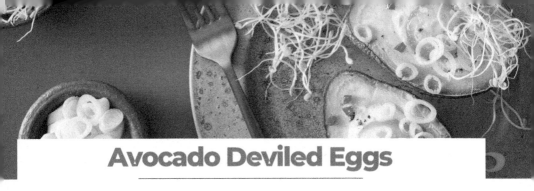

Avocado Deviled Eggs

INGREDIENTS

- 6 eggs, hard-boiled
- 1 ripe avocado
- 1 tsp mustard
- 1/2 lemon, juiced
- Salt and pepper
- Paprika

PREP. TIME: 20   SERVINGS: 6

DESCRIPTION

A twist on classic deviled eggs, using creamy avocado instead of mayo, garnished with paprika for a touch of spice.

DIRECTIONS

1. Peel and halve the eggs, removing yolks to a bowl.
2. Mash the yolks with avocado, mustard, lemon juice, salt, and pepper.
3. Spoon or pipe the mixture back into the egg whites.
4. Sprinkle with paprika.
5. Chill until serving.

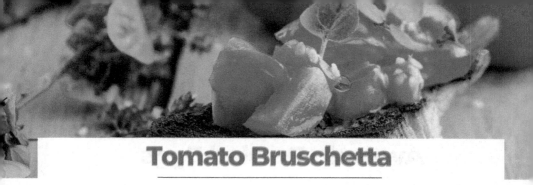

Tomato Bruschetta

INGREDIENTS

- 4 slices of rustic bread, toasted
- 2 tomatoes, diced
- 1 clove garlic, minced
- 1/4 cup basil, chopped
- 2 tbsp balsamic vinegar
- Salt and pepper
- 2 tbsp olive oil

PREP. TIME:
10

SERVINGS:
4

DESCRIPTION

Classic Italian bruschetta with a mix of chopped tomatoes, basil, and balsamic, served on toasted slices of bread.

DIRECTIONS

1. In a bowl, combine tomatoes, garlic, basil, balsamic vinegar, salt, and pepper.
2. Drizzle olive oil over the toasted bread slices.
3. Top each slice with the tomato mixture.
4. Serve immediately for a fresh and tasty snack.

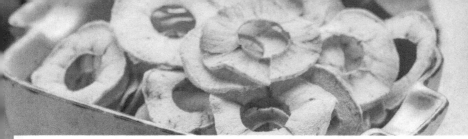

Baked Apple Chips

INGREDIENTS

- 2 apples, thinly sliced
- 1 tsp cinnamon
- 1 tbsp sugar (optional)

PREP. TIME: 10

SERVINGS: 2

DESCRIPTION

Thinly sliced apples, baked until crisp and lightly dusted with cinnamon, a sweet alternative to traditional chips.

DIRECTIONS

1. Preheat oven to 200°F (90°C).
2. Arrange apple slices in a single layer on a baking sheet lined with parchment paper.
3. Sprinkle with cinnamon and sugar if using.
4. Bake for 45 minutes, turning halfway through, until crisp.
5. Cool before serving.

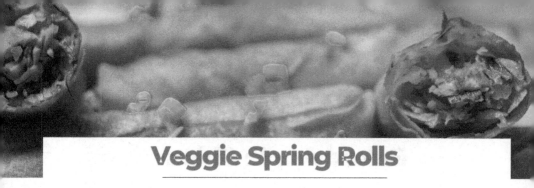

Veggie Spring Rolls

INGREDIENTS

- 8 rice paper wrappers
- 1 carrot, julienned
- 1 cucumber, julienned
- 1 bell pepper, julienned
- 1/4 cup fresh mint leaves
- 1/4 cup vermicelli noodles, cooked
- Dipping sauce (hoisin, peanut butter)

PREP. TIME: 20   SERVINGS: 4

DESCRIPTION

Fresh vegetables and vermicelli wrapped in rice paper, served with a tangy dipping sauce.

DIRECTIONS

1. Dip rice paper wrappers in warm water until soft.
2. Lay out on a clean surface and place a mix of carrots, cucumber, bell pepper, mint, and vermicelli on each.
3. Roll up tightly, tucking in the sides.
4. Serve with dipping sauce.

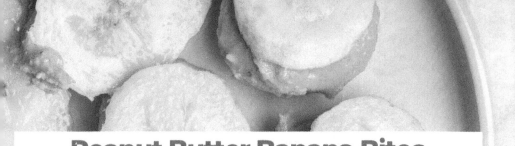

Peanut Butter Banana Bites

INGREDIENTS

- 2 bananas, sliced
- 1/4 cup peanut butter

PREP. TIME:
10

SERVINGS:
4

DESCRIPTION

Slices of banana sandwiched with peanut butter and frozen, a quick snack that's both sweet and satisfying.

DIRECTIONS

1. Spread peanut butter on a slice of banana.
2. Top with another banana slice to make a sandwich.
3. Freeze for at least 1 hour.
4. Serve cold for a refreshing treat.

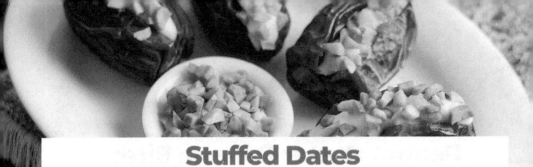

Stuffed Dates

INGREDIENTS

- 12 Medjool dates, pitted
- 1/2 cup almond butter
- Sea salt

PREP. TIME:
10

SERVINGS:
4

DESCRIPTION

Medjool dates stuffed with almond butter and sprinkled with sea salt, a deliciously sweet and nutty snack.

DIRECTIONS

1. Fill each date with almond butter using a small spoon.
2. Sprinkle a little sea salt on top of each.
3. Chill in the refrigerator until ready to serve.

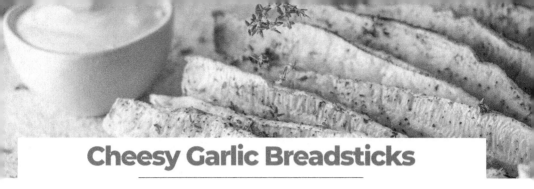

Cheesy Garlic Breadsticks

INGREDIENTS

- 1/2 lb pizza dough
- 2 tbsp butter, melted
- 2 cloves garlic, minced
- 1 cup mozzarella cheese, shredded
- Marinara sauce for dipping

PREP. TIME: 15   SERVINGS: 4

DESCRIPTION

Soft, cheesy breadsticks flavored with garlic butter, perfect for dipping in marinara sauce.

DIRECTIONS

1. Preheat oven to 375°F (190°C).
2. Roll out pizza dough and cut into strips.
3. Mix melted butter with minced garlic and brush over dough strips.
4. Sprinkle shredded cheese on top.
5. Bake for 10 minutes or until golden and cheese is bubbly.
6. Serve warm with marinara sauce.

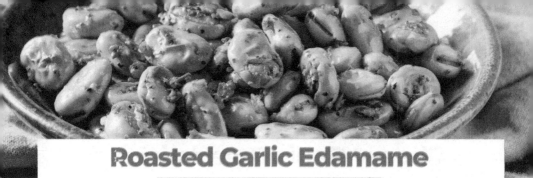

Roasted Garlic Edamame

INGREDIENTS

- 2 cups edamame, shelled
- 2 tbsp olive oil
- 3 cloves garlic, minced
- Sea salt

PREP. TIME: 5

SERVINGS: 4

DESCRIPTION

Edamame beans roasted with garlic and sea salt, a protein-rich snack that's both tasty and heart-healthy.

DIRECTIONS

1. Preheat oven to 375°F (190°C).
2. Toss edamame with olive oil, minced garlic, and sea salt.
3. Spread on a baking sheet in a single layer.
4. Roast for 10 minutes, until lightly golden and crispy.
5. Serve warm or at room temperature.

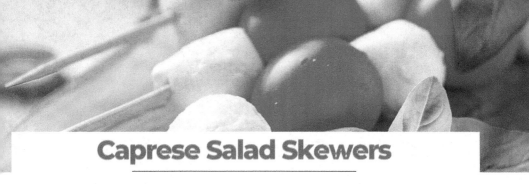

Caprese Salad Skewers

INGREDIENTS

- 16 cherry tomatoes
- 16 small mozzarella balls
- 16 fresh basil leaves
- Balsamic glaze

PREP. TIME: 10   SERVINGS: 4

DESCRIPTION

Cherry tomatoes, mozzarella, and fresh basil leaves drizzled with balsamic glaze, served on skewers for an elegant snack.

DIRECTIONS

1. Thread a cherry tomato, a basil leaf, and a mozzarella ball onto each skewer.
2. Repeat until all ingredients are used.
3. Drizzle with balsamic glaze before serving.
4. Serve chilled or at room temperature.

Carrot Cake Energy Bites

INGREDIENTS

- 1 cup rolled oats
- 1/2 cup grated carrot
- 1/2 cup dates, pitted and chopped
- 1/4 cup pecans, chopped
- 1/4 cup coconut flakes
- 1 tsp cinnamon
- 1/4 tsp nutmeg
- 1/4 cup honey

PREP. TIME: 15   SERVINGS: 12

DESCRIPTION

No-bake energy bites made with grated carrots, oats, and spices, mimicking the flavor of carrot cake without the guilt.

DIRECTIONS

1. In a food processor, combine oats, dates, pecans, coconut flakes, cinnamon, nutmeg, and honey.
2. Pulse until mixture is well combined and sticky.
3. Stir in grated carrot.
4. Roll mixture into small balls.
5. Refrigerate for at least 1 hour to set.
6. Enjoy as a bite-sized snack.

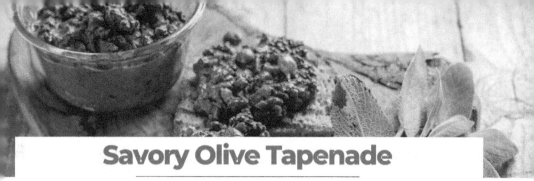

Savory Olive Tapenade

INGREDIENTS

- 1 cup mixed olives, pitted
- 2 tbsp capers
- 1 clove garlic, minced
- 1 lemon, zested and juiced
- 2 tbsp olive oil
- Fresh parsley, chopped

PREP. TIME: 10

SERVINGS: 4

DESCRIPTION

A rich and savory olive tapenade spread, ideal for pairing with crackers or as a dip for vegetables.

DIRECTIONS

1. In a food processor, combine olives, capers, garlic, lemon zest, and juice.
2. Pulse until finely chopped.
3. With the processor running, slowly add olive oil until the mixture becomes a coarse paste.
4. Stir in chopped parsley.
5. Serve with crackers or sliced vegetables.

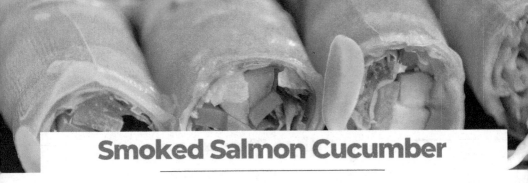

Smoked Salmon Cucumber

INGREDIENTS

- 1 cucumber, thinly sliced lengthwise
- 4 oz smoked salmon, sliced
- 1/4 cup cream cheese
- Fresh dill, for garnish

PREP. TIME: 15

SERVINGS: 4

DESCRIPTION

Thinly sliced cucumbers wrapped around smoked salmon and cream cheese, garnished with dill for a refreshing snack.

DIRECTIONS

1. Lay cucumber slices flat on a clean surface.
2. Spread a thin layer of cream cheese on each slice.
3. Top with a small piece of smoked salmon.
4. Roll up tightly.
5. Garnish with dill.
6. Serve immediately or chill before serving.

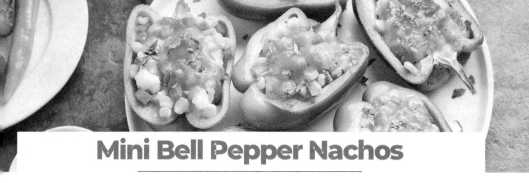

Mini Bell Pepper Nachos

INGREDIENTS

- 10 mini bell peppers, halved and seeded
- 1 lb ground turkey, cooked and seasoned
- 1 cup cheddar cheese, shredded
- Sour cream and salsa for serving
- Fresh cilantro, for garnish

PREP. TIME: 10   SERVINGS: 4

DESCRIPTION

Mini bell peppers sliced and loaded with seasoned ground turkey and cheese, a low-carb alternative to traditional nachos.

DIRECTIONS

1. Preheat oven to 375°F (190°C).
2. Arrange bell pepper halves on a baking sheet.
3. Spoon cooked ground turkey into each bell pepper half.
4. Top with shredded cheese.
5. Bake for 10 minutes, until cheese is melted.
6. Serve with a dollop of sour cream and salsa.
7. Garnish with cilantro.

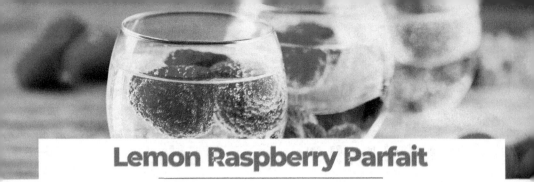

Lemon Raspberry Parfait

INGREDIENTS

- 1/3 cup chia seeds
- 1 1/2 cups almond milk
- 2 tbsp lemon juice
- 1 tbsp lemon zest
- 1/4 cup honey
- 1 cup fresh raspberries

PREP. TIME: 15

SERVINGS: 4

DESCRIPTION

A refreshing and light parfait layered with lemon-infused chia pudding and fresh raspberries.

DIRECTIONS

1. In a bowl, mix chia seeds with almond milk, lemon juice, lemon zest, and honey.
2. Stir well and let sit for 5 minutes. Stir again, then refrigerate for at least 2 hours or until it achieves a pudding-like consistency.
3. To assemble the parfaits, spoon a layer of chia pudding into glasses, followed by a layer of fresh raspberries.
4. Repeat the layering process until all ingredients are used.
5. Serve chilled, garnished with a few extra raspberries and a sprinkle of lemon zest.

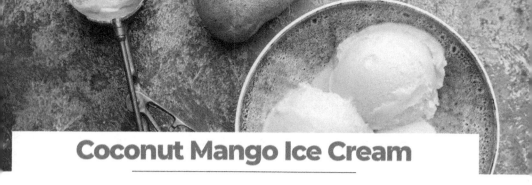

Coconut Mango Ice Cream

INGREDIENTS

- 2 cups mango, chopped and frozen
- 1 can coconut milk
- 1/4 cup honey
- 1 tsp vanilla extract

PREP. TIME:
10

SERVINGS:
6

DESCRIPTION

Dairy-free coconut mango ice cream that's creamy and tropical, perfect for a hot day.

DIRECTIONS

1. In a blender, combine frozen mango, coconut milk, honey, and vanilla extract.
2. Blend until smooth.
3. Pour the mixture into an ice cream maker and churn according to the manufacturer's instructions.
4. Transfer to a freezer-safe container and freeze until solid, approximately 4 hours.
5. Serve with additional mango pieces or a sprinkle of coconut flakes.

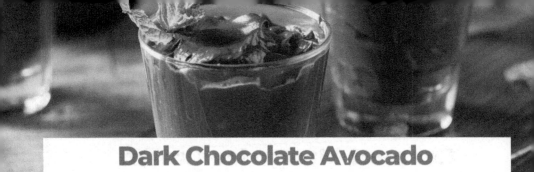

Dark Chocolate Avocado

INGREDIENTS

- 2 ripe avocados
- 1/2 cup dark chocolate, melted
- 1/4 cup cocoa powder
- 1/4 cup honey
- 1 tsp vanilla extract

PREP. TIME: 10

SERVINGS: 4

DESCRIPTION

A rich and silky mousse made from avocado and dark chocolate, offering a healthy twist on a classic dessert.

DIRECTIONS

1. Melt the dark chocolate in a double boiler or in the microwave, stirring until smooth.
2. In a food processor, blend the avocados until smooth.
3. Add the melted chocolate, cocoa powder, honey, and vanilla extract to the food processor.
4. Blend until all ingredients are well combined and the texture is creamy.
5. Spoon the mousse into serving dishes and refrigerate for at least 1 hour.
6. Garnish with a sprinkle of sea salt or a few chocolate shavings before serving.

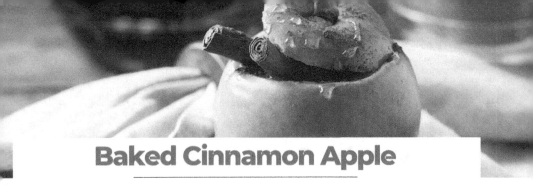

Baked Cinnamon Apple

INGREDIENTS

- 3 apples, thinly sliced
- 2 tsp cinnamon
- 1 tbsp sugar (optional)

PREP. TIME:
10

SERVINGS:
4

DESCRIPTION

Crispy apple chips baked with a dusting of cinnamon, perfect for a healthy, sweet snack or dessert.

DIRECTIONS

1. Preheat oven to 200°F (90°C).
2. Line a baking sheet with parchment paper.
3. Arrange apple slices in a single layer on the baking sheet.
4. Mix cinnamon and sugar, if using, and sprinkle over the apple slices.
5. Bake for 1 hour, flip the slices, and continue baking for another hour or until the apple slices are crisp.
6. Cool completely on a wire rack before serving to allow them to crisp up further.

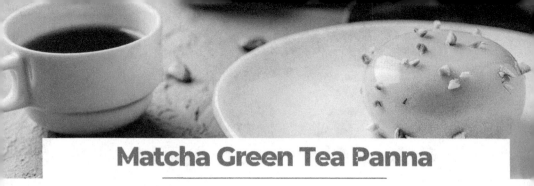

Matcha Green Tea Panna

INGREDIENTS

- 2 cups heavy cream
- 1/4 cup sugar
- 1 tsp matcha green tea powder
- 1 tbsp gelatin
- 1/4 cup water

PREP. TIME: 15   SERVINGS: 4

DESCRIPTION

A creamy panna cotta infused with matcha green tea, providing a delicate balance of sweetness and earthy flavors.

DIRECTIONS

1. In a small bowl, sprinkle gelatin over water and let sit for 5 minutes to soften.
2. In a saucepan, heat heavy cream and sugar until the sugar dissolves and the mixture is hot but not boiling.
3. Whisk in the matcha powder until fully incorporated.
4. Add the softened gelatin to the matcha mixture and stir until the gelatin is completely dissolved.
5. Pour the mixture into molds or serving glasses.
6. Refrigerate for at least 4 hours, or until set.
7. Serve chilled, garnished with a light dusting of matcha powder.

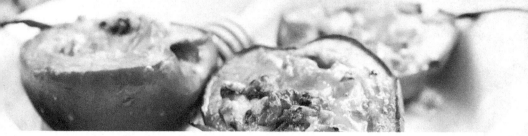

Walnut-Stuffed Pears

INGREDIENTS

- 4 pears, halved and cored
- 1/2 cup walnuts, chopped
- 2 tbsp honey
- 1/2 tsp cinnamon
- 1/4 tsp nutmeg
- Butter

PREP. TIME: 10   SERVINGS: 4

DESCRIPTION

Tender baked pears filled with a sweet and crunchy walnut mixture, drizzled with honey.

DIRECTIONS

1. Preheat oven to 375°F (190°C).
2. Place pear halves on a baking dish, cut side up.
3. In a small bowl, mix walnuts, cinnamon, nutmeg, and a little butter.
4. Fill each pear half with the walnut mixture.
5. Drizzle honey over the stuffed pears.
6. Bake for 25 minutes, or until the pears are soft and the filling is bubbly.
7. Serve warm, perhaps with a scoop of vanilla ice cream or a dollop of whipped cream.

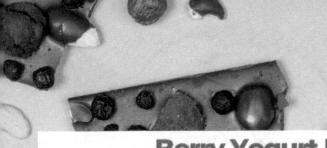

Berry Yogurt Bark

INGREDIENTS

- 2 cups Greek yogurt
- 2 tbsp honey
- 1/2 cup mixed berries
(blueberries, raspberries)
- 1/4 cup granola

PREP. TIME:
5

SERVINGS:
4

DESCRIPTION

Frozen Greek yogurt bark topped with fresh berries and a hint of honey, a refreshing and colorful treat.

DIRECTIONS

1. Line a baking sheet with parchment paper.
2. Mix Greek yogurt with honey, then spread evenly on the prepared sheet.
3. Sprinkle mixed berries and granola over the yogurt.
4. Freeze for at least 3 hours or until completely firm.
5. Break into pieces and serve immediately or keep frozen in an airtight container.

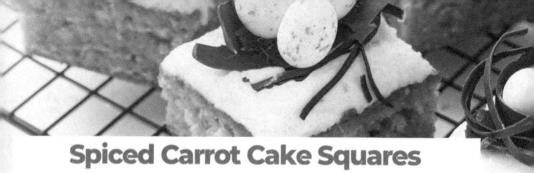

Spiced Carrot Cake Squares

INGREDIENTS

- 2 cups grated carrots
- 1 cup flour
- 1/2 cup sugar
- 1/2 cup applesauce
- 2 eggs
- 1 tsp vanilla
- 1 tsp cinnamon
- 1/2 tsp nutmeg
- 1/2 tsp baking soda
- Frosting: 1/2 cup cream cheese, softened
- 1/4 cup powdered sugar

PREP. TIME:
15

SERVINGS:
12

DESCRIPTION

Moist and flavorful carrot cake squares, spiced with cinnamon and nutmeg, topped with a light cream cheese frosting.

DIRECTIONS

1. Preheat oven to 350°F (175°C).
2. In a large bowl, mix flour, sugar, cinnamon, nutmeg, and baking soda.
3. Stir in eggs, vanilla, and applesauce until well combined.
4. Fold in grated carrots.
5. Pour batter into a greased baking dish.
6. Bake for 30 minutes or until a toothpick inserted in the center comes out clean.
7. Cool completely.
8. For the frosting, beat cream cheese and powdered sugar until smooth.
9. Spread frosting over cooled cake.
10. Cut into squares and serve.

No-Bake Peanut Butter

INGREDIENTS

- 1 cup peanut butter
- 3/4 cup graham cracker crumbs
- 1/4 cup melted butter
- 1/4 cup sugar
- 1 cup chocolate chips

PREP. TIME: 15

SERVINGS: 12

DESCRIPTION

Easy no-bake peanut butter bars with a chocolate topping, a satisfying treat that combines sweet and salty flavors.

DIRECTIONS

1. In a bowl, mix peanut butter, graham cracker crumbs, melted butter, and sugar until well combined.
2. Press the mixture into a lined square baking dish.
3. Melt chocolate chips in the microwave or over a double boiler.
4. Pour melted chocolate over the peanut butter base.
5. Refrigerate for at least 1 hour, or until the chocolate sets.
6. Cut into bars and serve.

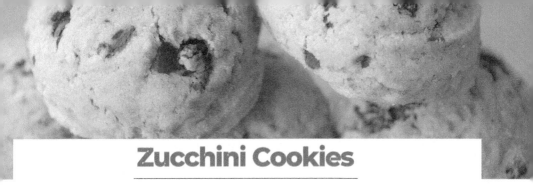

Zucchini Cookies

INGREDIENTS

- 1 cup shredded zucchini
- 1 cup all-purpose flour
- 1/2 cup brown sugar
- 1/2 cup unsalted butter, softened
- 1 egg
- 1 tsp vanilla extract
- 1/2 tsp baking soda
- 1/2 tsp salt
- 1 cup chocolate chips

PREP. TIME:
15

SERVINGS:
24

DESCRIPTION

Soft and chewy cookies made with shredded zucchini and chocolate chips, a sneaky way to include veggies in a dessert.

DIRECTIONS

1. Preheat oven to 350°F (175°C).
2. In a mixing bowl, cream together butter and sugar.
3. Beat in the egg and vanilla extract.
4. Stir in shredded zucchini.
5. In another bowl, whisk together flour, baking soda, and salt.
6. Gradually add dry ingredients to the wet mixture, mixing until just combined.
7. Fold in chocolate chips.
8. Drop spoonfuls of dough onto a baking sheet lined with parchment paper.
9. Bake for 12 minutes or until golden brown.
10. Cool on a wire rack before serving.

90-DAY MEAL PLAN

Tips for Success

Accurate Portion Sizes: Use measuring cups, spoons, and a kitchen scale to ensure portion sizes are accurate. This accuracy is crucial for keeping within the calorie limits specified in the meal plan.

Preparation Is Key: Prepare meals in advance whenever possible. Meal prepping helps you stick to your diet plan and avoid the temptation of opting for less healthy options when you're hungry.

Stay Hydrated: Drink plenty of water throughout the day. Sometimes, thirst is confused with hunger. Keeping hydrated can help manage hunger and aid in weight loss.

Customize to Your Taste: Feel free to swap out certain ingredients based on your dietary restrictions or preferences. However, ensure to keep the calorie count approximately the same to stay within the meal plan guidelines.

Monitor Your Progress: Keep a food diary or use a mobile app to track your meals and calories. Tracking what you eat can be an effective way to ensure you're following the meal plan correctly.

Listen to Your Body: Pay attention to how your body responds to the diet. If you feel consistently sluggish or hungry, you may need to adjust the meal timings or portion sizes slightly. Always consult with a healthcare provider before making significant changes to your diet, especially if you have underlying health conditions.

Adjusting the Plan

Not everyone's body reacts the same way to a specific diet plan. Here are a few adjustments you might consider:

Adding Variety: To prevent dietary boredom, rotate different recipes within the same calorie range. Variety can help you stay motivated and committed to your diet plan.

Incorporating Exercise: If you are able to exercise, you might need slightly more calories to compensate for the energy expended. Consult with a healthcare professional about adjusting your calorie intake when incorporating exercise into your routine.

Your Plan

If you want to print your plan, follow the instructions belo. Otherwise move to the next page

1. Open your camera app

2. Point your mobile device at the QR code below

3. Download and Print the plan

Made in the USA
Las Vegas, NV
16 September 2024